WEIGHT LOSS SURGERY

The Practical Guide to Coping with Post-Surgery Emotions

Michael Beck

© Copyright 2017 Michael Beck

All rights reserved.

The information in the following pages is broadly considered to be a truthful and accurate account of facts and as such any inattention, use or misuse of the information in question by the reader will render any resulting actions solely under their purview. There are no scenarios in which the publisher or the original author of this work can be in any fashion deemed liable for any hardship or damages that may befall them after undertaking information described herein.

Additionally, the information in the following pages is intended only for informational purposes and should thus be thought of as universal. As befitting its nature, it is presented without assurance regarding its prolonged validity or interim quality. Trademarks that are mentioned are done without written consent and can in no way be considered an endorsement from the trademark holder.

Table of Contents

Introduction 5

Chapter 1: Emotional Decisions........................... 7

Chapter 2: Mind over Matter 13

Chapter 3: Real Life Stories 19

Chapter 4: Choosing Surgery Options 37

Chapter 5: Post-Surgery 52

Chapter 6: Bariatric Surgery for Children? 59

Conclusion.. 62

Discussion 64

Introduction

Congratulations and thank you for downloading this book. I hope you will find the information you are looking for and can apply this information to your plan for weight loss.

In the following chapters, we will discuss the journey of what obese individuals go through in the struggle to be mentally and physically healthy and accepted. All they want is a life that isn't filled with depression and hatred; to be able to enjoy going out into the world and not be ridiculed for having the disease of being overweight. You will experience their thoughts and feelings as they begin their plans for the last chance; that is weight loss surgery and how to *deal with the aftershock.*

There are plenty of books on this subject on the market, thanks again for choosing this one! Every effort was made to ensure it is full of as much useful information as possible. Please enjoy!

With many people behind you, you will grow in strength with each day and have renewed hope that this time, your plan will work and your life will be turned around in many positive ways. It just takes time, and you have that time now. Move forward and don't look back until you have completely succeeded in where you want to be. Keep a journal so you can then see where you were and where you are today; enjoying life for the first time.

Thanks again for downloading this book, I hope you enjoy it!

Chapter 1: Emotional Decisions

Over an estimated 200,000 people every year elect to have weight loss surgery. But, even though people are proud of their accomplishments and transformation, it was a very difficult journey. The emotional consequences are many. Realizing the extreme negative health issues, ridicule, and severe sadness and depression drives them to make a final and major decision to seek weight loss surgery. Accomplishing their goal of weight loss is their only hope of ever having a happy and normal life and getting rid of this terrible disease once and for all. One filled with hope, and happiness; feelings that some have never had, and others have experienced but are missing now. Most of these people want help but are very fearful of it for lack of information.

A woman in her sixties tells about how proud she was after her surgery. She worked hard to get to the healthy weight and appearance she now has. While the transformation is amazing, not only because she looks great, but how she has maintained her plan with exercise and a low-calorie healthy diet, she now faces the emotional trauma yet again; a very different problem than she was facing before surgery, but trauma nonetheless. Now, she has better health, and her energy has dramatically improved. She shows tremendous confidence; confidence that was long missing in her life since childhood.

She finally reached out to her family, who have been trying to help rid her of this disease by suggesting healthy alternative only to have her turn away from them. Like other debilitating issues such as alcoholism, the patient has to finally reach that end-of-the-road point themselves (you can lead them, but you can't "make them" get well). Her family was relieved when she came to them, and they were able to discuss a plan without animosity but with hope instead. She talked them into just one more final try and one more diet just to make sure and she gave this challenge everything she had but again failed. Mentally, it was the last straw for her, and now she was up to the challenge. It was time! They researched options together, locating specialists in bariatric surgery and making appointments with a couple of the best professionals they found. Also in their plan, they thought it was important to get some professional psychotherapist assessments to prepare for this huge change.

Since having her weight loss surgery, she lost half of her weight in approximately eight months and continued to lose more weight each month at a steady pace; she was able to maintain her weight while eating a healthy diet and is building her body as well with plenty of exercises. She has an abundance of energy, and her family is very proud as well.

Because this is a life-altering decision for people suffering from obesity, it may take years before they are ready for weight loss surgery. Her family talked about it, and friends offered to help, but they had to tread very lightly on this subject. It was really like walking on eggshells, and fearing their loved one and friend would withdraw even more emotionally, because of the frightening thought of the actual surgery. They are also fearful of whether or not they might be too fat and not make it through a surgical procedure. They could actually die on the operating table. What if it doesn't work? It could be the answer, but maybe not, and they feel even more confused and withdrawn. Eventually, that seed that was planted in their brain from family and friends, about a possible solution, is starting to grow.

Still, it is the threat now of moving out of their miserable, and yet safe "comfort" zone and into the frightening thought of surgery. Most people when they reach the point of researching surgery as a last resort, have been on multiple diets and low calorie, low carbohydrate diets. They will lose a few pounds, only to keep gaining it back and most often they will gain more weight than when they started their plan. After several years, they discover they suddenly are faced with health problems such as headaches, backaches, hip and knee problems, and eventually these issues lead to more serious signs of health problems like energy levels dropping; signs of diabetes and hypertension; and signs of possible heart problems.

It is highly recommended that prior to having weight loss surgery; you should consult with a bariatric psychotherapist who specializes in weight loss surgery consultation. It is suggested that you also try to find doctors who have a holistic approach. Your general physician can recommend a specialist for you and even a bariatric surgeon. Most often these two specialists will have offices and in the same building and possibly the same medical company. After you have some names of professionals, you can then research online for their accreditation and reviews. Also, ask your physician if he has any reference he can share with you who have had bariatric surgery and can share their experience with you.

You should also join some support groups. If you do this before your procedure and with enough time before surgeon, it will be an unbelievably positive boost for you heading into this plan. Try to locate an exercise physiologist and a dietitian. Both can help further your plan not only before your surgery but after. At some point, it might be necessary to lose a few pounds prior to surgery for a successful outcome.

Then make appointments. Start first with the psychotherapist because that is the doctor who will help you deal with the emotional unknowns of the surgery and will be able to answer all of your questions prior to your procedure and afterward to establish realistic goals and anticipation to learn to manage new resulting changes. This is a very important part. Those who think they are ready and just decide they know what they are doing and what it is all about are just tricking their mind into thinking it isn't necessary.

After discussions with this specialist, it is time to move on to the next phase of your plan. Contact an excellent bariatric surgeon. Look for one who has all qualities such as excellent bedside manner, spends a lot of time with you, explains everything in ways you can completely understand, carefully goes over everything with you, and has reviews of the best doctor in the whole world, plus is young, single and gorgeous! If you happen to find a doctor with all of those qualities, you are the only one who has. These specialists are unique. They operate for hours sometimes on tiny areas of the stomach. They should have a lot of the qualities but not all. I would rather have a professional that has poor bedside manners and is a highly successful surgeon who is current with all of the newest techniques and equipment and has been specializing and performing bariatric weight loss surgeries for a lot of patients who are all desperate to fix their broken lives. People have said that the time when they are being admitted to the hospital just before surgery, is the most difficult time. The anticipation is immense, and your mind is out of control with negative and positive thoughts at the same time. When you are prepared, and the surgeon arrives to give you the assurance that he will take good care of you, which will be difficult because it is now the reality. It is not easy, and your team, family friends, doctors, and nurses know that. They are compassionate and will get you through it.

The following are brief descriptions or explanations of the four different weight loss surgery procedures. Your weight loss surgeon will give you more details, but this will give some basic information. The first three are the most preferred by doctors and patients, and the fourth procedure is only performed in a matter of severe obesity with health problems.

Chapter 2: Mind over Matter

Obese people are obsessed with their cruel and depressed existence. They think about it constantly. It is on their mind, and it is all they think about. They feel they are going to break into a million pieces and really wish with all they have, that they would just get it over with and explode. Get it out of their head.

Severely overweight people are always on the edge of a major breakdown. All of this turmoil happens when they're alone. They go to bed, and they think and think and think and can't sleep because their mind is a mess with questions, messages, thoughts and dark depression and terror. Then they wake up, and it's still there looming over them like a huge buzzard waiting to snatch their prey. These are things that constantly travel in and out of a severely depressed and overweight person's mind. There seems to be a padlock on their brain, and they can't find the key. It overpowers them and puts the failure and shame right in front of them. Some of this turmoil is expressed below in the thoughts of an obese woman:

There is disappointment everywhere I turn. I have disappointed everyone, even myself. Friends and family want me to participate in special events but I can't. I don't feel like it.

I want to go outside and into the garden and sit on the bench in the shade, but I can't. My legs won't let me. They are large; so large that I can't see my feet to move.

I have nothing to wear. Even my underwear doesn't fit. I don't want to buy new things until I lose all my weight, but I have nothing to wear.

I am miserable in my bed. I can't move or roll over. My body hurts with pain all night. It keeps me awake.

I want to take a shower and wash all of this fat and skin down the drain, but I wish I could just fit. If I could wash myself away and disappear, I would. It takes so long to shower. I just sit on a large bench in my oversize shower made especially for me. I sit and let the water pour over me. I don't want to move.

Is it time to eat breakfast? This time I won't eat. I will starve myself and not eat anything. I wonder how long it takes to starve my huge obese body! I hate the word, "obese" but that's me.

Why didn't my mother and father help me when I was little? Why did they let me have anything to eat that I wanted? Why did mother tell me that before I could leave the table, I had to eat everything on my plate? Why did my father tell us that if we ate everything, we could have ice cream?

I would like to go out to a restaurant and eat sometime, but I can't because people stare and share disgusting remarks with each other. I know because I can almost hear them. I hate people who whisper.

I do want to wear makeup someday, but it wouldn't help. I am ugly, and I can see that in the mirror. I had the mirror. Someday it will be gone!

I open the curtains just a little and take a peek outside. I don't like the sun really. I like it at night more. I used to like the sun, but I don't really.

My feet hurt. They always hurt. I wonder if thin people's feet hurt. My toes are so ugly; they are obese. I have very fat toes. I would wear socks, but I can't put them on.

How did I get here? I just always remember being Fat. I want to cry but I can't anymore. I just can't.

I can still live alone, but people have to bring me things. They don't bring me things that will help me though. Not usually.

I am trapped! This is me and this is who I am. I hate ME! I am afraid to die.

People with obesity are very good at telling lies. They will lie to themselves by blaming everyone and everything around them for their disease. It is either the food in the restaurant or because parents were obese and it is just in the genes. Sometimes it is just because other people are cooking the meals and they don't consider your severe weight problem, or Grandma does, but she feels good when you eat her dinners she brings over.

Have you ever been to a family reunion and you see a relative that you haven't seen in years? That relative looks great. He looks very much the same as he did years ago. When asking him how he kept in shape all those years he said that he had always watched his weight and through diet and exercise he can maintain his weight and energy. This is most likely what you did not want to hear, and so you retreat into hiding in a corner by yourself until all family has left. The truth is hard to hear. Even though some people will not directly mean to hurt you, it hurts nevertheless.

When you endure direct hurtful messages, they then start to make you angry, but that anger is more feelings of shame than anger. Then shame can start thoughts of fixing the problem. That is certainly the hard part. How? When? Can I fix it or is it too late? It is only too late when you die. Starting early than later will give you a much better and happier life in the long run. There will be those bumps in the road, but they are not large enough that you can't climb over them.

There are many tools you can use before you are ready to decide.

Self-honesty is a great a beginning too. Stop lying to yourself and others. Learn to face your fears. This has probably been the number one issue and is at the top of your "Stop/Think" list. When you are truthful, it will seem strange to hear words you do not want to hear, but it is essential in healing and moving forward.

Get organized by preparing the necessary tools for research; such as a calendar, computer to research, journal, pens, paper, folders, and books on Weight Loss Surgery. Then you are ready to start a pre- and post-surgery nutrition and exercise plan. Before having bariatric surgery, try to construct a set of guidelines that you can use for healthy eating, exercises, and a healthy lifestyle.

Chapter 3: Real Life Stories

The following are some stories that people have written about their journeys through the process of being fat to obese.

I am a young woman of twenty-six, named, Ginny. I have been overweight since I was about ten. My issues with food started after my mom died suddenly with a heart condition that we didn't know she had. No one knew, not even dad. I am the one who discovered her. She was a wonderful stay-at-home mom. We lived in a fifteen-room historical home built by Frank Lloyd Wright. I was born just after our family moved in. My dad was a builder and had his own small construction business. My grandparents lived not far from our home.

I had twin brothers and an older sister who took care of me when mom went shopping or to garden tea parties. Mom never worked inside or outside of our home because we had cleaning people came over every Tuesday.

I had a happy childhood. I guess you'd say it wasn't normal because we had everything. We were spoiled but not in a bad way. We learned respect, kindness, and above all never to tell lies. My sister was married when I was five. She was fourteen years older, and I was her flower girl. I look back at Polaroid photos of myself and my brothers. I still love the curly edges of the instant photos that peel away from the film, but I hate the photos. I hide them, but every once in a while, I get them out. Not often though, because I looked adorable with my sweet little dresses and my long curly hair. I had an innocence about my smile. My dresses were just above my knees, and you could see my skinny legs with patches of bruises from playing and climbing trees with the boys. And my shoes were shiny black with straps across the front that covered my white lace socks. I can remember like it was yesterday. Mom took the photos, and that is the only reason I get them out of the closet to look at. I see my eyes looking at my mom. Happy eyes, but not now.

I was just 10. Excited about getting home from school because Saturday was my birthday and mom had made a special cake. I ran through the front door of our house calling for her. I dropped my art paper by the stairs. I bent over to pick it up, but it was stuck on the strip of wood near the landing, and it tore. I made it for mom. It was a cartoon of the kids that will be at my party. I had a very funny feeling. I remember it and still experience that feeling from time to time. It was like a sweet flower smell from a puff of air. For some reason, it took my breath away for a second.

I stood up and called again. Mom was usually near the door to greet us from school. The boys were older and went to a different school, so they were a while longer getting home. I liked that because I had mom all to myself for a while.

I called again and started to search the rooms for her. Since I could smell the cake, I went to the kitchen. The cake was decorated and oh, so special. It was my favorite chocolate cake with pink candles. Mom was not there. Calling, I went room to room. The last room I went to, I noticed the door was open a crack. Mom loved that room because it was quiet and she could get away from the noise and read a while. It was the last room at the end of the hall near the back stairway. I saw her there on the floor. She was not moving when I whispered to her. I was quiet; I was frozen, I could not move. Fear, hurt, anger, sadness and an enormous amount of grief came into my tiny body. "Mom?" I picked up her beautiful glasses with the "diamonds" in the corners and look them all over to see if they were broken. I picked up her book; then I looked to see if her stomach moved to see if she was breathing but she wasn't. I touched her hand it was cold. I screamed; screamed so loud it seemed like it was for an eternity!

Mom died of a sudden heart attack. There were no warnings. Life was in a suspended hole, and I just wanted to stay there. This was when my "eating" problems began. I blamed mom for a long time for leaving us. She never saw my art, but that's okay. It was torn. I trashed my room my dad said, but I don't remember that. My pick quilt that mom maid at quilting circle is somewhere in my closet. I don't want it. I hate that thing.

I have a lot of anger, and because of that, I have gained so much more weight now, but I don't care. It just doesn't matter to me or anyone. I didn't care then either; I ate that damn chocolate cake. I took it to my room and hid it, and ate it. I am no longer a sweet, cute little girl who looked like my mom. I hate my existence, I do want to even live, but then, I love my food. I live alone now, and that is just what I like.

My sister comes to visit and brings me food. She tried to get me to eat "special" things that she makes. I have been on every single diet there is. I even tried to starve myself again, but it didn't work. Nothing works. I am so fat now that my feet and legs won't hold me up for very long because I am just plain tired. I have stopped blaming mom for all of this and would like to get better. I think sometimes; I feel that she is talking to me. I can hear her voice. She is telling me, "Don't give up. Be strong. You can do it. You are my special girl." I even dreamt about my mom recently. She was holding my paper, and I could see she taped it." I woke up and cried. I need help. I will do this for mom.

It was my dad who helped me when I called. We talked for a long time. He brought information about surgery techniques when just dieting won't do the job. We researched together and made a list of doctors and made appointments. Dad is going with me.

I am afraid!

It's Christmas, and our family is here. Every one of them I think. It is very crowded. I am Earl, and I am FAT!! In fact, everyone in the family is fat. I was actually born fat, so I really don't know what it is like to be a "normal" weight. I weighed almost twelve pounds when I was born. My mother had a lot of trouble having me she said because of her large size. My mother weighed almost four hundred and eighty pounds. She had to have a cesarean, but due to her weight, it was very dangerous. She had other issues as well. She had diabetes, and that is what really ended her live years later but I think it was the combination of having the disease and being obese (there's that word I hate to use) but that's what it is.

A few days after Christmas, my mother and father and my brother, sister and I, made our usual three times a week trip to the grocery store. Mother and Father always had trouble getting into the car even though it was a van, so that took a while before we were on the road. We didn't have far to go but had to go through our busy little town. We were probably a sight to see because looking out of the window; I saw that people were actually not only staring but pointing and laughing; laughing out loud, and my father was mad. He was going to get out of the car and beat the tar out of them. But my mother said to just ignore them; that they don't know us.

We arrived at the Piggly-Wiggly grocery store (oddly enough it was the only store in our small little town). I loved going to the store. It seemed we spent hours in there and had several carts we were loading up with food and such. My brother and sister and I did not even have to ask if we wanted something. Food was cheap there. We had different jobs to pick out certain items. First on my list were cookies. Since Oreos were my favorite, I put about six packages of those in the cart. We got home with a mountain of groceries! Our van was packed to the ceiling.

After unloading, of course, everyone was starving. We always snacked first then mother would cook up something great with mashed potatoes and gravy, fresh baking powder biscuits, brown sugar squash, green bean casserole, chicken and rice casserole, and hot dogs in case we didn't want chicken. Then we ate a huge amount of desserts. This was our normal routine, and we made at least three trips to the store each week. Our mother loved to cook, and we all loved to eat.

It was when I was in my senior year of high school that life's reality hit me like a ton of bricks.

I needed someone who actually cares about me. Senior Prom and no one would accept my invitation, not even the ugliest girl there. I was hurt and miserable. I started fasting, but that didn't work. I started eating a little less, but that didn't work. I went on Weight Watchers, but that didn't last. In fact, I kept on gaining. My brother and I still have races to the kitchen to get what's left of a meal. We never, ever have leftovers.

I was miserable for several years after that and stayed home and out of sight. I am handicapped because I am so overweight and have difficulty walking. I can't work either. It is difficult to get work when you are severely overweight. It is my brain more than anything. I received low-income benefits and assistance. I always tried to use humor to cover up my food addiction; making fun of myself and people like me. But it is not funny anymore. I want what my friends have. I want a good life, with a family and I don't want to marry an obese person even though like me, they need to be loved. But they need to find help like I am doing. I have a friend who will help me find a doctor who specializes in weight loss surgery. I don't want to have diabetes the rest of my life.

Wish me luck! But I will do this anyway.

I am sixty-six years old, and my name is Connie. I have been large or overweight for about twelve years. I have a good job, still employed and working for the city offices in a mid-size community. My husband, John, retired a couple of years ago. He is not very overweight but maybe just a little. We have been married for about thirty years. My husband and I have been having some angry disagreements for a while now, and I think it is due to my weight and his retirement. It wasn't an issue before he retired and we managed fine; only have some minor issued like most married couples have. But now it is much worse, and I am afraid of losing him.

John has given me an ultimatum that if I don't make serious attempts to lose weight, he was leaving. He has hurt me with his criticism, calling me disgusting and lazy even though, I am the one working. I get out of the house, but it is difficult.

Two years ago, I had to have a pacemaker installed to keep my heart regulated. I also have a serious liver disease and had pancreatic surgery to remove two small cysts that thankfully were benign. But unfortunately, they had to remove my spleen at the same time, and now my immune system is compromised, so I have lots of colds and flu. I am always sick it seems.

I have researched and talked to a surgeon about the possibility of having weight loss surgery. The best option for me would be having this surgery. My doctor explained about the high risks of surgery with as many serious conditions that I have. There is only one option, and I am very afraid although I seem to like this doctor and have confidence in him. I am going to proceed with my research. I do not want to lose John, and I feel it is all my fault. I feel so terrible all the time and think that might even be making him mad. We don't go anywhere like we use to or even sit down at the table at the same time. He picks at me for the amount of food on my plate so now I am eating small portions then after he goes to bed, I eat the leftovers. I am so ashamed.

I have so many questions to ask besides the risks. I just want to be a good wife and do the right thing for us. The thought of living alone is far worse than the surgery.

-Connie-

My name is Patty, and my story really began when I was sixteen. I am thirty years old now. I have been overweight most of my life just because I love to eat. I love the smell and taste of food. I grew up with a parent (my father) who was a chef at a popular restaurant in Columbus, Ohio. He was amazing, and I was always in the kitchen at home, or sometimes I could sneak into the restaurant (they would let me in the back door). My mom worked as a checker at a specialty meat store. My dad loved the fresh meat she would bring home at his request via written list he would give her every other morning. He never bought meat too far ahead and never froze it either. He said that destroys the flavor of meat and fish. I loved to assist him. He taught me about the history of food and spices and showed me how to use them together. We would set aside one night a week where we would use different items in the kitchen refrigerator, spice drawer or vegetable bin to create a special dinner without a recipe.

It was a wonderful life, but as a consequence, I was a very fat child. My parents, however, were not. They were healthy and fit. My dad was a runner too. He would get up early, grab a big glass of cold milk, drink it and then run. He did not drink coffee because he just said it was bad for your health. My parents were really not concerned about my heavy body but thought that it was just baby fat that I would lose when I grew up. My father loved to watch me eat because he knew I loved food.

I had a lot of friends and most were overweight too, but not as fat as I am. I really didn't care. Sometimes we could share clothes, and that was fun. We had a group of five of us. We went everywhere together, and we were happy. We were bullied and made fun of, but because we were all together, it didn't matter. One time when I was about thirteen, one of my friends told me she was moving to another state because her dad was being transferred. We were all so sad to have a part of us leave. We promised each other that we would always be there for each other and that even though far away, we would connect.

A few months after she moved, there was a football game that the four of us planned to attend, but it was in a different town about twenty miles away. One of my friend's older brothers, who drives, said he would take us. It was okay with all of our parents. He was a good driver and responsible. It was on Friday night, four days away. On Thursday, I happened to be at the park on my way home from school when I started down a long stairway. I tripped and fell down about six steps to the bottom cement. I was taken to the hospital where I was diagnosed with a concussion. So, obviously, I had to break the news to my friends that I would not be able to go.

Tragically, on Friday night my friends lost their lives in a very bad traffic accident. It was reported that a car traveling the wrong way on a double lane highway and crashed into three vehicles and there were no survivors. This event was so devastating that it sent me into a tailspin of "why I am alive, and my friends are not" depression. I had many years of counseling. That is nothing you can ever get over, but I have learned to live with it even though I am not the same person I was. I could barely come out of my room, so my dad brought me comfort foods to my room. I lived under a blanket with the shades drawn for months. I absolutely could not deal with life anymore. Being fat and unable to walk some days didn't help. I made a bed in my closet and took my cat, (crinkle) in with me. I did not want company and did not want to be seen. My dad would put a tray right by the closet door for me. I felt like I was my own prisoner with a tray brought to me and having it slid in a long cold metal opening (that really wasn't there), but I felt like it was. Daddy meant well though.

I had to go to school but dreaded it every single day. It seemed like I had the Plague the way the kids stared at me and called me names. Where was the compassion? I just lost my friends for heaven's sakes. They stuffed their leftover food in my backpack and in the cracks of my locker. I was isolated. I just knew that if I looked in that mirror again, I would see plastic wrap covering my whole body. It was a horrible existence. My grades went down, and mom and dad wanted me to go to counseling yet again. Another shrink is going to tell me what? Nothing, that's what? He isn't me and doesn't know about me at all.

I kept in contact with my other friend who moved away, and we wrote back and forth a lot. She recently told me that she had weight loss surgery and is on the road to recovery and has a great new outlook. She is engaged and wants me to come to her wedding in about eight months. She is really losing the weight and is excited.

Even though it will be difficult to give up all of the food that I so joyously love to eat, I want to pursue having the same surgery she had. She is sending me lots of information and even invited me to stay with her after my surgery so she can teach me her healthy diet plan and show me the exercises she is doing.

I wanted to be a chef; because of my dad. I think now it is good that I didn't go in that direction. I could never live up to my dad's amazing meals. I might just become a writer. I think about my angel friends and know they are with me and also Sara. We miss them terribly. I believe in fate, and I was protected that tragic Friday night. Everyone has a path that is placed in front of them that they walk down. I believe that. People come and leave, but some people stay. I am glad my friends were there for a while. That was such a gift to me. I am so lucky.

So, now I am thirty, and this is where my real fantastic story will begin. I am really excited each time I look in the mirror and tell that person that life is better than this. And I let her know that the exterior of that person I see (and of course, some of the interiors) needs to go.

My mother and father will be proud of me, I know. I am picking myself up and walking forward! I can do this, especially if my best friend can. Maybe I will meet some special person and invite her to my wedding.

Goodnight my angel friends!

This is "our" weight loss surgery story. There are two of us who will be going through this together because we are identical twins, Robert and Ronnie. We have always been very close and think the same things. We like the same things too, but something about us is very different. We are twenty-eight years old. Born on Valentine's Day. Our picture was in the local newspaper. Most people could not tell us apart but our mom could. I am Robert and am starting this story on paper for you. We had a great childhood most of the time. We fought but only in fun. I am 6'4" and so is Ronnie. We both had dark hair and blue eyes. Our difference is that I weigh 180 lbs., and Ronnie weighs 360 lbs. So, now people can tell us apart. Ronnie has diabetes, but thankfully I do not.

I am Ronnie. I hate myself, but Robert cheers me up. We have separate lives but not far from each other. I am married and have two children. My rapid weight gain only happened about four years ago, but I have had diabetes for more than six years. After a couple of years of putting off getting tested for to find out why I was just not feeling well, I decided to go ahead to try to get a diagnosis. I was sure though that it had to do with my diabetes and I was afraid it would open a whole can of beans that I didn't want to be opened. It was actually my wife who talked me into it for the "sake of the kids." I had a lot of issues and worries. I was depressed, cold all the time, muscle cramps, and tired, very tired. As I had started to gain weight, it seemed that I really wasn't eating that much to cause all this weight. The tests always came back negative for anything except low in iron.

After searching, I found a specialist who was highly recommended. His special was Internal Medicine, but he was great! After the first consultation, I knew that I connected with him and he was great at answering and asking questions. I learned a lot from him. He said he wanted to run some testing of his own. He wanted to rule out things but first had a hunch that it might be thyroid related.

That is the test he ran, and sure enough, that is the culprit. I am on my way to feeling great again. The doctor did mention that I might look into the least invasive weight loss surgery due to my large size. He said it is easier to put weight on than take it off and it would be better for diabetes and to prevent and heart or lung issues to get the weight off and keep it off. He gave me referrals to the specialist that he knew who would be excellent to talk to see if, in fact, that would be the best option. They may decide on a healthy diet and exercise program instead but that it would be best to talk to them.

My wife is extremely relieved to know that the condition can be fixed. If I had waited though, until other more serious symptoms occurred, it would not have been easy. Plus, my weight was a major concern to my new doctor. Someday in the not so distant future, I am looking forward to playing ball with my boys.

Here I am again to tell you that I am as excited for him as I can be. We have been extremely worried, but the road to recovery isn't quite over. We have faith. I, too, am married to my grade school sweetheart. We have four kids now, and life is good.

It is important to have family support. We are there for my brother, and maybe someday people won't be able to tell us apart anymore.

R & R

Chapter 4: Choosing Surgery Options

Gastric Sleeve Bypass

The **Gastric Sleeve Surgery** is next popular weight loss surgery procedure. If a patient has a high body weight index (BMI), this surgery is less risky. People who have severe weight issues with major lung problems, heart conditions, liver or intestinal problems your physician will advise another surgical method to use that will be much safer and better for the patient.

Gastric Sleeve surgery is used as an assistant to weight loss and is probably the most important procedure for people with high BMI numbers. Your doctor will place you on a restricted diet prior to this type of surgery to prepare your much smaller stomach for less food intake. You will be required to follow this diet as prescribed for the best outcome.

During this surgery, almost seventy-five percent of a patient's stomach will be removed; leaving a narrow gastric tube, also called the "sleeve." The part of the stomach remaining is long and narrow, resembling the shape of a banana. It will keep its new longer shape. This type of surgery is meant to keep patients intake amounts of food to a limited level, so the stomach will only be able to process those smaller amounts, resulting in a faster feeling of being full. The patients will feel many times they are not hungry after this surgery. Hence, the stomach is smaller and fills up faster. Another positive result of this procedure is that a hormone found in the stomach called, ghrelin, (which causes the hungry feelings) is now very minimal because most of it has been removed with the rest of the stomach.

The duration of the gastric sleeve surgery usually takes one to two hours and is performed using a laparoscopic procedure where the surgeon will make two to five incisions in your stomach. The surgeon then uses a camera, scope, and instruments, working through the incisions to remove the section of the stomach. The stomach is stapled then with surgical staples, and the cuts are closed with stitches.

The benefits of this procedure are that it is a simple solution to weight loss, with a fairly quick recovery time. The Gastric Sleeve procedure is less invasive, making it a shorter surgery time than the other procedures, and time of healing and recovery is drastically reduced. There are no other organs involved in this operation, and fewer medications are needed. This surgery has had remarkably positive results. There is very little care required, and very few patients complained of complications or adverse side effects. Your weight loss will be gradual over the next two years, but that is better and easier on your body than if you remove weight too fast.

Following your surgery, your diet will consist of clear liquids only. It may be hard at first, but many patients have had minimal food cravings right after surgery. After the first week, you can add foods like pudding, Jell-O, ice cream, and yogurt.

After a few more weeks, soft foods can be added to your diet; then after one month you should be able to eat any healthy foods, but they should still be soft foods. Your physician will be giving you a more complete healthy diet plan.

The Gastric Sleeve surgery is the best surgical procedure for overweight patients to achieve weight loss using surgical intervention. This procedure was first performed almost thirty years ago, but it was a much more invasive surgery then. New and better techniques have drastically improved, and this has become the number one procedure of all gastric surgeries with very few complications reported. It has been proven to have a high success rate in patient's weight loss expectations. The result for patients is they feel with their physician's help, had made the right choice. Patients report that because of this surgery their overall health has improved dramatically plus they have succeeded in losing the weight they wanted, and that is a healthy weight. Their energy is back, and they feel great! They are working hard to maintaining their new life with healthy diets and plenty of exercises, and are very encouraged and proud. Family and friends can see the hard work and continue to be by their side. It was a difficult journey but well worth it in the long run. They do not look back but concentrate on working to keep healthy, plus most are helping others that had similar or the same story. The feedback from patients who have completed this surgery and those who have succeeded in their journey are encouraging to medical research and the information gathered will also help others to face their fears about bariatric surgery.

In the first three years after surgery, patients will see a dramatic result in their overall weight loss. Patients weight loss should average at least seventy percent of their excess weight during this time. A significant advantage also is that the patient will see improvements to their overall health that had affected high blood pressure, diabetes, depression, and anxiety. It is important to continue to follow up with your psychotherapist to make sure that things are still on track.

Some patients may opt to have the gastric sleeve surgery initially, and then when they have lost some of their excess weight, they will go ahead with a second procedure called, "gastric bypass." The combination surgical plan is for patients with lower BMI (Body Mass Index) resulting in even greater excess weight loss, more than average.

Some patients preparing for the Gastric Sleeve surgical procedure may find that sometimes when surgery has been completed; the surgeon had changed this procedure to the Gastric Sleeve instead. If during surgery, he finds a considerable amount of scar tissue or other concerning problems that place the patient at more risk, he will make the decision immediately to proceed with the gastric sleeve technique instead of this riskier gastric bypass technique.

For those people who have very high BMI, this procedure can be used as part of a longer approach to weight loss. Because it is less risky for these patients, it can be used a year or two before a gastric bypass is performed. People who are high-risk patients are often the ones who receive this procedure because of the risk factor being lower than other, more invasive, techniques.

Patients, who have serious lung disease, heart disease, or intestinal disease, often have this operation because it is faster and has a lower risk. This procedure is best also if a patient is a senior age. During surgery, if the doctor finds considerable amounts of scar tissue, he may opt to make a change to another procedure instead. The use of a gastric bypass procedure will be less risky to the patient.

Your physician will explain this in more detail. Next, we will explain Gastric Bypass surgery.

Gastric Bypass Surgery

Gastric Bypass Surgery has been used longer than all other bariatric procedures for weight loss. This procedure will significantly decrease the size of your stomach; even more than the gastric sleeve. It is a major surgery that will leave you tired and hungry but will only be able to have liquids. Like any surgery, you will be tired and uncomfortable. The good news is that the negativity will pass. Any surgery has some difficult issues. One very important thing is to walk as much as you can after surgery as it will ease the pain.

The way this surgery works is that the surgeon will be removing a small section of your intestines and he will re-route remaining organs and tissues in your digestive system. Recovery time for this procedure has a lot to do with the size of the incision the surgeon makes; either laparoscopic where several small incisions are made, and the physician can use instruments and cameras to work or using a large open incision. Either way, you will be required to stand and walk some after surgery to remove any trapped gas left over from using air to inflate your abdomen to make it easier to work around the stomach area.

The gastric procedure works because food that leaves the smaller stomach will turn into waste and will bypass most of the large intestines. This technique minimizes your fat absorption to reduce the amount of calorie intake from the food you eat. Patients will experience more and faster weight loss in a short period of time. People who have more serious health issues such as diabetes or heart disease early in life, or struggling with severe obesity issues, the gastric bypass surgery is needed to avoid more major health issues.

Your surgeon will add vitamins and minerals to your diet prior to and after surgery. Gastric bypass surgery has some downsides though. By rerouting large and small intestines, your body's ability to absorb natural and healthy food vitamins will be reduced, and that is why extra vitamins and minerals will be required.

A drastic change in diet will be necessary starting a few weeks before surgery and maintaining a good healthy diet. If you are eating foods that have high grease content and fatty foods as well, you will develop negative side effects like having diarrhea and vomiting, along with the terrible gas and indigestion that goes with it.

After the patient is discharged, usually two or three days after surgery, they will feel a little frightened that they are by themselves. The family should be asked to be there when the patient returns home.

Gastric Band Surgery

Patients who opt for the Gastric Band surgery, or "Lap-Band," must adhere to the physician's strict dietary specifications. Also, they would not be a candidate for this surgery if they had intestinal disorders or if they are regularly taking aspirin because of the involvement of the stomach and intestines.

Gastric band surgery involves the placement of a small soft silicone ring that the surgeon places at the top part of the patient's stomach. This ring has an inflatable balloon in the center that is used later to inject saline into it. When the ring is in place, the stomach then has been divided into two sections; a very small section on top above the band, and a larger part of the stomach on the bottom. After a person eats, food enters and fills the small section on top so less food and calories can enter. After a few hours, the food makes its way through a hole in the ring and then begins digesting normally.

After the ring is in place, the surgeon then places a port under the skin that is attached to the ring using soft, flexible tubing. The port is then used to add or remove saline which will inflate the balloon that separates the two parts of the stomach. When saline is injected into the expander, it will expand the balloon making the area between the two stomach divisions smaller so less food will enter and the patient will feel very full, and the process of passing the food between the two sections will be a very slow process. When saline is removed or decreased, it will pass larger food particles through faster.

This procedure is a preferred surgery because it will help them feel full sooner and for a longer amount of time. There is a common side effect that can occur, and that is the band can slip up or down from where it is initially placed. This can affect your weight loss success. What if this happens? There are a lot of systems to look for if this happens. Let your surgeon know if you experience sudden abdominal pain; changes in eating as if you were able to eat more without feeling discomfort, or the opposite and not being able to eat much at all; vomiting or nausea as you may have the feeling of something caught up or trapped and you want to throw it up; or you could experience acid reflux where gases are coming up through your esophagus.

If you have any of the above and feel that they are unusual occurrences, you should notify your surgeon as quickly as you can. He will then be able to make some adjustments to put it back in place.

It might just be a matter of deflating the band so that it will fall back into its original position. If this can't be done, a follow-up operation might be required to reposition it or even band removal. No one wants to experience this or even have to have an additional surgical procedure, but if it needs to be removed, the surgeon can go over other options for you.

Benefits of this type of surgery are that almost a fifty percent excess weight loss occurs after surgery. The improvements to health conditions are remarkable. The procedure is less invasive than most, and your hospital stay will be decreased with very short recovery time. As long as you stick to the healthy diet and exercise plan, your health will be drastically improved, and your energy levels will be high. Also, your mental awareness sharpens, and you will have self-confidence. It is just as important if not more important to have a better mental outlook. Everyone around you will notice the difference.

Now, after surgery, your doctor is going to want you to eat healthy food and exercise more. Stay positive and look ahead not back. You had a rough life, but you are on the road to a great new life. You will feel like you have been born again. Get involved with family and friends. Make new friends by joining groups. Support groups would allow you to tell your story and help others through these difficult struggles. You will be amazed at your special journey and accomplishments. You will be very proud!

Biliopancreatic Diversion Surgery

The last weight loss surgery listed in this book is the Biliopancreatic Diversion Surgery which actually has two different techniques. One includes the Duodenal Switch. A surgeon will only perform this weight loss surgical procedure if the patient is extremely obese and their weight is causing such serious health problems that could result in death. This procedure is used only as a last resort. To be a candidate for this surgery, a person must be severely obese. Their body mass index has to be at least fifty or higher.

So, here is some information about the other procedure, the Biliopancreatic Diversion. This surgery is a type of gastric bypass surgery that is rarely done due to its complexity. It is a high-risk major surgery that can actually cause serious health issues due to resulting in less absorption of food. The procedure involves using general anesthesia, then rather than using small incisions (laparoscopic) as in other bariatric surgeries a large open incision is made, removing a large portion of the stomach; then the portion that is left (or small pouch), is connected to the lower part of the small intestine. The small intestine is separated in its center rather than the lower part; the lower section of the small intestine is joined to the stomach pouch; reattachment of the two sections of the small intestine is reattached down near the digestive tract. This surgery is usually performed by making a large incision. In some cases, the surgeon can operate using the laparoscopic procedure.

Depending on which technique the surgeon used, you will have to be careful to avoid too much exercise and just rest in order to heal faster. It will be advised to rest for the first two weeks. The diet will be an all liquid diet for a while, and a lot of rest will be required. Normally, it takes about six weeks to resume some normal activity. The physician will give your further instructions concerning your meal planning as far and what to eat and how much, plus what medications you will be prescribed. Your surgery will leave you with an iron deficiency, as well as vitamin and mineral deficiency. As a patient feels better, they will be advised to attend counseling and support groups to help them to stay positive. This is a difficult surgery not only physically but mentally as well. Recovery depends on the support and good positive attitude.

Some of the risks of this surgery have been reported as infection, fluid leakage into the stomach area, peritonitis, iron deficiency, diarrhea, nausea, shaking, unsteady, deep vein thrombosis, pulmonary embolism, gallstones, anemia, constipation, and osteoporosis. Your surgeon will advise before choosing this surgical procedure, any complication issues.

For the first few weeks after surgery, you will be eating very small amounts of food, because of your new stomach size. They will be mostly liquids and soft foods. It will be important to drink small amounts of water throughout the day to stay hydrated.

You will feel a full feeling a lot faster and will not absorb many calories during this time. Usually, during the first year, you will notice a significant decrease in weight. The expectations vary with each individual.

Listen carefully to your surgeon because it will make your recovery easier and more successful. He will give you specific instructions to follow for diet and exercise. You do not want to have this happen again. Be aware of that on any of the surgeries. Your doctor is a major component in your success.

Bariatric surgeries range between twenty thousand dollars and thirty thousand dollars.

Chapter 5: Post-Surgery

For some reason, life after bariatric surgery seems to threaten some people. Jealousy plays a part in problems that come up. Sometimes a spouse will suddenly feel threatened, and disagreements will start arguments. Some people have to seek marriage counselors to get through the hard times. It shouldn't be like that. Spouses will usually feel a need to take care of someone who is in dire need of feeling wanted but instead feels depressed and lonely. A spouse will wait on their loves one hand and foot, but when they don't have that need, they will get angry and alone. Friends sometimes will have jealousy also. Maybe they are struggling some in their life, but before your successful outcome, they could lean on you, and they felt safe. They could cheer you up, and it made them feel great, but now things have changed.

These emotional things will take time and patience. You will have that but in time. You have to concentrate on getting to the end of that tunnel, and they will have to understand. You are fixing what was wrong with you, and they will have to do the same.

Parents and grandparents who saw you, and now are looking at someone unfamiliar, and they don't know how to handle that. They might make snippy remarks because it is hard for them to deal with. You can teach them. They need to just look into your eyes to see that you are there and even better.

Some people who are in horrific accidents or return from serving in the military have terrible debilitating injuries. These people are the same in their soul, but they have to work hard to prove to their loved ones that they are the same person, only better because they have gone through a journey similar to yours that gives them courage, love, compassion not fear, anger, and depression. You will receive support from others that you would never have expected.

Some family members, such as her mother, and siblings, made hurtful remarks ("I don't understand why she had to do that. I would have tried other options besides surgery.") held only a passing effect.

Emotional issues can appear out of nowhere. You might have major mood swings. Some people might be very angry one minute because they step on the scale and see they have gained ten pounds. That is all they can see. They don't think about the two-hundred eighty-five pounds they have lost. It makes them so angry that they see failure again. Sometimes they look at themselves in a mirror when they get up in the morning, and they are looking at the old image before even starting a weight loss plan. It truly is a roller coaster for a while.

Painful memories take a very long time to heal. Unfortunately, they never go away, but they fade after time. It is a fact though, that after surgery people still remember their deep, painful existence before that, they still try to hide. They tend to want to stay home and read or just watch a movie and not be noticed. This is really the most difficult time because it is the time when loneliness creeps back in, and you tend to reach for food. Another important thing to remember after surgery is not to have anything but healthy food in your home. In time, you will come out into the world, but it's okay for a while. Your friends can really help at this point. Even have a get-together at your place. Serve healthy snacks and beverages. When you have lost a lot of weight, the compliments can sometimes make you feel uncomfortable. Obese people suffer for years. That is literally years of abuse. It is really all that you knew. No wonder it takes much time to get through it.

Comfort food is hard to forget. It has been left behind but not forgotten. To overweight people, it is the beginning of their miserable life, and yet they miss it. One woman said it was the "devil" in her deviled cake. But that was her favorite. Dinner out is one of the worst things people who are overweight or beginning to gain extra pounds attributed most of that to eating out.

People who live alone will not want to cook for themselves, and after working all day are too tired to stop at the store for groceries and then go home to cook. If they do that, then most of the time after getting home, they are too tired to cook, so they go back out and grab a burger and fries at their favorite fast food restaurant. They might call a friend and meet for dinner out or even any time of the day. It is so nice to relax with friends and eat out, have a glass of wine and dessert too. After all, if any extra you will have dinner the next night too. Not only are these really poor eating habits with a huge number of calories, but expensive as well. Then to top it off, when you arrive home you are way too tired to exercise.

Other health conditions a person has are at risk by eating out, especially if they have had any heart surgery. That glass of wine just might send them to the hospital. They order the wine, but no one knows that bringing that wine out to them that they are not supposed to have it.

When eating out with friends, another problem is that friends like to coax you into eating things you shouldn't. "Oh, just take a bite of my caramel ice cream cake. A little taste won't hurt you; you have lost so much weight. Besides, this is the best dessert I have ever tasted in the world." With friends like that, who needs enemies? A really good friend would never do to you what is not right and put you in a bad spot of having to refuse.

Losing huge amounts of body weight causes a lot of physical changes. Changes that are not comforting at all and really are discouraging. It is another problem that you have to knock off of your list. One by one the problems will disappear. Extra hanging skin will be embarrassing as well as debilitating. And yet, another doctor enters your life when you have to seek a plastic surgeon. Some people just hide the extra skin with large clothing but usually end up filling the sagging skin with fat again. It is the disgusting part of weight loss surgery, but it can be remedied. New techniques for cosmetic surgery are popping up all the time. Make sure to get a doctor that is up on new ways to perform these surgeries and get names of patients that doctor has performed difficult surgery on so you have a reference.

Some plastic surgeries might not be covered under your insurance plan. Call your insurance company to get information. There are exceptions though, and they come in the form of health reasons. Do the research and again talk to people who have had this done. An example might be if an obese patient lost so much weight that they have skin folds hanging so low that it is difficult for them to walk around.

Studies show that for some people psychological problems are most common after weight loss surgery. From depression to alcohol abuse which can lead to binge eating and bulimia. These conditions can happen, but the instances are low. Most people were found to have a more enjoyable and healthy life after surgery.

Make sure you have kept your diary of your journey up to date. Keeping notes of your emotional adjustment, and the hurdles you have had to leap over is always there to remind you of the accomplishments and the changes you have made. Also, writing down changes in your diet and exercise with be amazing to look back on. Following your doctor's orders and making changes according to his plan for you is good to have written down. Your doctor may change medications from time to time or schedule follow-up visits to go over all of your questions and concerns. Keep track of everything you can in your book.

Meditation is something many people do, and it clears your mind to make room for new thoughts. It also relaxes and refreshes your mind. Document everything about your journey so you can reflect back to remember your strength.

Life moves forward, and your struggles and surgery are left behind. You have strength and courage to do what it takes to keep going forward, and you will have a longer and richer life now that you have walked down that path. Some things are just a bump in the road. People choose whether to walk over the bump or leap over it. Choose "LEAP!" Choose to walk forward and don't look back on all of the tough times. Put your head up and say, "I did this, and I am proud!"

Chapter 6: Bariatric Surgery for Children?

Children suffering from obesity is becoming more common each year. Obesity in children is at high risk for contracting diabetes, type 2. In fact, they are at risk for the same diseases seen in obese adults. These children have a high probability of being morbidly obese when they are an adult.

When children are diagnosed with obesity, they are thoroughly evaluated and depending on the test results, everything possible to be done in order to avoid surgery will be made. It is imperative to treat these diseases in children quickly to avoid the serious consequences in contracting other health issues.

There are a few cases that non-surgical options are not as effective as surgery is. Every child's situation is different, and you may be referred to a pediatric surgeon. You will need to work together with the surgeon to make the best plan for your child that will be the best outcome. Sometimes you may not be able to work with an individual surgeon and will have to seek a second opinion to get the confidence you need from him to move forward. This plan will involve life changes for both you and your child, also family and friends. It's entirely different for an adult, but when it is your child; your protective mode is on guard. When you have your child's team in place, you and your child will have to follow a very strict plan. This is a very difficult time when child surgery is performed. You will receive a healthy eating and exercise plan for your child before acceptance is made for your child.

After a child is accepted for obesity surgery, the actual surgery will become the key element that will assist in the overall plan for a healthy weight loss to improve your child's life. This surgery is looked at as a long-term and necessary part of the overall plan. It is not an easy thing to do. Usually, the failure of this plan is in managing it.

There are very few of these procedures done. There are discussions of a moral issue and the consequences later that can deter people from resorting to such drastic measures on children that do not understand or can speak for themselves. An incident a few years ago was reported where they subjected a two-year-old to gastric bypass surgery. He was extremely overweight, and the extra fat was actually causing him to have breathing problems. It is for this reason that bariatric surgery should only be performed in severe emergency situations. Teens that are overweight also should be involved in nutrition classes where trained professionals can assist in a weight loss program. It is well worth the month and the price instead of subjecting a child to weight loss surgery.

If surgery is found to be the last resort as in the case of the two-year-old boy, then all caution must be given. If the child is facing surgery that child must be prepared if old enough to understand the outcome and effects when he gets home after surgery.

Normally, a lap-band or gastric bypass is performed. These surgical techniques are usually performed using a laparoscopic method. The patient will be in the hospital two to three days to make sure there is no infection. That is the highest risk, especially for children.

After being discharged and home, special care should be taken to keep your child from high activities. Bands do slip occasionally and a second surgery may be necessary to readjust the band or remove it. Your pediatrician will provide you with diet and exercise plans and how to care for the wounds.

Conclusion

Thank you for making it through to the end of this book. Let's hope it was informative and able to provide you with all of the tools you need to achieve your goals whatever they may be.

You really have to be dedicated. Don't put it off; this is a chance you have finally found that will change your life and make it amazing! You will be doing this not just for yourself but for your family and friends as well. Get informed, ask questions, do research and above all, stay focused. Bariatric surgery is not a complete solution, but it's the tool that will help you get there.

You will no longer have fears and feel ashamed. You will feel special, loved and respected by people you would not even know yet. The specialists and medical professionals and so many others will care for you and journey with you as you leap over that bump in the road. Even though very difficult, it is do-able!

Your team of medical professionals will make sure the steps you are taking are the right steps for you. Not everyone making this choice will require the same steps or the same procedures. Your life will be changed forever.

After the surgery is over you will have a new mindset. You will be able to realize that you have to "eat" for different reasons, and not because you are ashamed of your fears or hiding behind your comfort food because you had feelings of failure, but because it is the only solution and you are ready! You will make this journey and you will be proud and maybe help others because you have been through it and made it!

Finally, if you found this book useful in any way, a review on Amazon is always appreciated!

Discussion

Questions You Might Ask?

Every person seeking weight loss surgery will have questions. Some are valid and should be asked, while others don't make any sense to people who are not obese. See some of the questions below that you might ask your surgeon.

After surgery, will my stomach remain small new size, or is it like loose skin that will become larger again if I eat a little more than I should? During surgery, some procedures remove part of it, and surgical procedures will divide it. Your stomach will do what it always has done; it will stretch in time by the amount of food you consume. If you stick with a healthy diet your nutritionist provides you or by your surgeon; it will remain the same. It can both enlarge and shrink.

Will I still have high blood pressure? Getting to a healthy size and weight does many things to the medical issues you have had. Your blood pressure can be controlled or even disappear with proper diet and exercise. It is diagnosed when other causes are present. Blood pressure is certainly raised, and most people with excessive weight problems will have it.

How soon will I have energy? When you are placed on a low-calorie diet and depending upon which surgery procedure is right for you, as you drop the weight and you are eating foods that are important for your health such as fresh green vegetables, your energy will start to get better. But you need proper exercise as well.

Will I die from weight loss surgery? It is rare but only at risk of death if you are extremely obese and has underlying major medical conditions; such as liver disease, heart disease; or has had heart attacks or intestinal disease. All precautions are taken by the team of professionals to keep you as safe as they can. You will constantly be monitored.

Will I have lot of pain after surgery? Everyone has a different amount of pain tolerance. Some will be uncomfortable for several days, and others may feel they need pain medications to get through the healing time. During surgery, you will be heavily medicated and will be given pain medication that will help for a couple of days. Your doctor is going to give you medication that will be reduced in amount each day, so you will able to get around. Exercise will be extremely important after surgery as well as nutritional supplements. Vitamins will be prescribed by your doctor, and it is important to follow his orders to the letter.

www.ingramcontent.com/pod-product-compliance
Lightning Source LLC
Chambersburg PA
CBHW060804260726

48660CB00002B/768